A
SECRET
TO HEALTH,
WEALTH,
PROTECTION
AND
HAPPINESS

BEN IJEOMA ADIGWE

A SECRET TO HEALTH, WEALTH, PROTECTION AND HAPPINESS
© 2021 by Ben Ijeoma Adigwe
ISBN:

Publishers:
Published in Nigeria by:
Nkanemi Services
www.nkanemi.com.ng
nkanemiservices@gmail.com
+2347051291988

Unless otherwise indicated, all scriptural references are from the Authorized King James Version of the Holy Bible.

TABLE OF CONTENTS

CHAPTER ONE

THE SECRET

There is a secret to health, wealth, protection and happiness to be found by a careful study of a couple of references in the Bible. It is to be found in the New Testament Book of 1 Peter 3:8-9.

> *"Finally, be ye all of one mind, having compassion one of another, love as brethren, be pitiful, be courteous;*
> *Not rendering evil for evil or railing for railing; but contrariwise blessing; knowing that ye are thereunto called, that ye should inherit a bless (KJV).*

The Amplified version of the above scriptures brings out the meaning more clearly. It says:

> *Finally, all [of you] should be of one and the same mind (united in spirit), sympathizing [with one another], loving [each the others] as brethren (of one household),*

> compassionate and courteous –
> tender hearted and humble-
> minded).
> Never return evil for evil or
> insult for insult – scolding,
> tongue-lashing, berating; but
> on the contrary, blessing-
> praying for their welfare,
> happiness and protection, and
> truly pitying and loving them.
> For know that to this you have
> been called, that you may
> yourself inherit a blessing
> [from God]-obtain a blessing
> as heirs, bringing welfare and
> happiness and protection.
> (1 Peter 3:8-9 Amplified
> version).

Verse 9 above rules out retaliation from our life experiences. It discourages retribution in our conduct with our fellow men. No evil for evil, or insult for insult. On the contrary you should bless your offender by praying for their welfare, happiness and protection and truly pitying and loving them. The verse goes on to say that to this kind of behaviour you have been called so that you may yourself inherit a blessing from God as His heirs; a blessing that will bring you welfare, happiness and protection.

The first blessing that will result from this non-retaliatory attitude that is prescribed is welfare. Welfare is defined in the dictionary as health, happiness, good fortune, well-being and prosperity. Well-being is further defined in the dictionary as the state of being comfortable, healthy or happy.

Thus, it can be said in the light of the above that your not taking a retaliatory stance would make you inherit a blessing from God to the effect that you would get good health, happiness, comfort, good fortune, prosperity and protection.

The above attitude of never rendering evil for evil was not Peter's original idea. It was rather what Jesus taught in His earthly ministry. He taught a lot on prayer but the first thing he ever said about prayer in the Gospels was this business of praying for our enemies. Hear him in Matthew 5:44:

> *"But I say unto you, love your enemies, bless them that curse you, do good to them that hate you and pray for them which*

despitefully use you and persecute you".

He went further to say that there is a reward for loving your enemies:

> "For if ye love them which love you, what reward have ye? Do not even the publicans do the same?" (Matthew 5:46).

Paul also spoke on this attitude of non retaliation in Romans 12:17.

> "Recompense to no man evil for evil. Provide things honest in the sight of all men".

> "Dearly beloved, avenge not yourselves, but rather give place unto wrath; for it is written, vengeance is mine; I will repay, saith the Lord. (verse 19)

> "Therefore if thine enemy hunger, feed him; if he thirsts, give him drink; for in

so doing thou shalt heap
coals of fire on his head.
(verse 20).

Admittedly, this is a hard attitude to adopt but it is absolutely necessary for a successful walk with God. Jesus Himself recognized the difficulty in adopting this kind of forgiving attitude so much that He said we should forgive a person 70 x 7 times if necessary (cf Matthew 18:22) i.e 490 times!

Jesus amply demonstrated this kind of attitude in his own life. Even on the cross he prayed to his Father to forgive those who crucified him (cf Luke 23:34).

The attitude of forgiving your enemies is a key to answered prayers and a successful walk of faith as Jesus taught in the Mark 11:25-26. There is no better way of demonstrating your forgiveness of your enemies than praying for their welfare, protection and happiness. Jesus said there was a reward for so doing. I believe the rewards that Jesus spoke of are those which Peter explained in 1 Peter 3:9.

CHAPTER TWO

THE SECRET TO WEALTH

Never return evil for evil or insult for insult – scolding, tongue-lashing, berating, but on the contrary, blessing – praying for their welfare, happiness and protection and truly pitying and loving them for know that to this you have been called, that you may yourself inherit a blessing (from God) – obtain a blessing as heirs, bringing welfare and happiness and protection 1 Peter 3:9.(Amplified version)

As noted before, one of the results of your not retaliating but praying for your enemies is that you yourself will inherit a blessing from God that would bring welfare. One of the dictionary's definitions of welfare is prosperity which is a state of being rich.

There are instances in the Bible of men who expressed this non retaliatory attitude and were stupendously blessed as a result. The character called Job in the Bible was recorded as being the greatest of all the men in the East (see Job 1:3). He was stupendously rich – the richest man in the East. He clearly had this attitude of non retaliation which contributed to his great wealth. We hear him recount his way of life in Job 31:29-30:

> *"If I rejoiced at the destruction of him that hated me, or lifted up myself when evil found him:*
> *neither have I suffered my mouth to sin by wishing a curse to his soul. (KJV)*
>
> *I have never been glad when my enemies suffered, or pleased when they met with disaster;*
> *I never sinned by praying for their death. Job 31:29 - 30 (Good news Bible Today's English Version).*

Job considered it a sin to curse him that hated him! No wonder he was so rich.

Incidentally, when he lost all his wealth during his trials, the Bible records that he recovered all and got extra when he prayed for his friends who spoke against him and accused him of evil doing.

> *"And the Lord turned the captivity of Job when he prayed for his friends: also*

Another Bible character that got so much wealth as a result of this attitude was Solomon. He had an encounter with God who appeared to him in a dream and asked him to ask for anything. He asked for wisdom from God.

God was so impressed, according to the account, that He replied that because he had not asked for riches, wealth, or honour, <u>nor the life of his enemies</u>, nor for long life, He (God) will give him riches, and wealth and honour, such as none of the kings have had before him or after him. (see 2 Chronicles 1:11-12). Solomon was one of the wealthiest men the world ever saw and one of those things that brought him such wealth, according to God, was that he didn't ask for the life of his enemies. No wonder Jesus said in His sermon on the mount that there is a reward for loving your enemies (Matthew 5:46).

Another character in the Bible who had stupendous wealth and power and who exhibited this godly character of non-retaliation was Joseph. In the Old Testament account of Joseph, his brothers hated him with a passion for his dreams and the extra favour that his father showered on him. They eventually sold him off as a slave and, by providence; he landed in Egypt and after much stressful, ugly experiences rose to become the Prime Minister of Egypt. All through his travails in Egypt before he rose to prominence, he never exhibited any iota of bitterness or resentment. Eventually, when he became the second man in Egypt and met his brothers again, he forgave them and sustained them. When his brothers feared that he would hate them and repay them with evil, the Bible records as follow:

> *"And Joseph said unto them, fear not: for am I in the place of God?*
> *But as for you, ye thought evil against me; but God meant it unto good, to bring to pass, as it is this day, to save much people alive.*
> *Now therefore fear ye not: I will nourish you, and your little ones. And he comforted them and speak kindly unto them"* *(Genesis 50:19-21).*

No wonder he was stupendously rich and powerful. It is a real food for thought that in the life of these three mighty and wealthy men of the

Bible – Job, Solomon and Joseph – this common trait
of not hating their enemies ran through them all.

CHAPTER THREE

THE SECRET TO HEALTH

As noted before, one of the benefits of not returning evil for evil is that we inherit a blessing of welfare, and happiness and protection according to the Amplified translation rendering of 1 Peter 3:9.

One of the dictionary definitions of welfare is Good Health. It is recognised even by medical doctors that hatred and resentment bring about a host of illnesses. A New York physician was reported to have said that 70% of his patients revealed resentment in their case histories. He said that ill-will makes people sick and that forgiveness will bring them good health better than many pills. The Christian doctor, Dr. S.I. McMillen in his seminal book, "*None of these diseases*", lists a host of diseases which are caused by anger, resentments and hatred.

There is also a case history of a patient who died as a result of a long held grudge which weakened his immune system. No wonder Jesus said there is a reward for loving your enemies in the Sermon on the Mount. One of such rewards, in the light of the above findings, is Good health. There is therefore a high cost for getting even.

In the parable of the unforgiving servant told by Jesus in Matthew 18:23-35, a king took account of his servants. One was brought to him who owed him about $10,000,000 (according to the Amplified translation). When he could not pay, his master ordered that he be sold with his wife and children and everything he possessed and payments be made. The servant begged that he be given sometime to pay. His master pitied him and forgave him the entire debt. But that same servant went out and found one of his fellow servants who owed him about twenty dollars (according to the Amplified translation) and he held him by the throat and said, "pay what you owe". The fellow servant begged him to give him some time and that he will pay him all. But he was unwilling and went and put him in prison till he should pay the debt.

When the behaviour of this servant was reported to the king, he was very angry and called him a wicked servant. He reminded him of his forgiving him because he begged him. He told him that he is expected to show mercy and forgiveness on his fellow servant as the king had mercy and forgave him. The master then in anger turned him over to tormentors, till he should pay all that was due unto him. Jesus rounded off the story by saying that this was how God will deal with every one who does not forgive his brother from their heart his trespasses.

The essence of the parable is that we offended God more than any person can offend us.

Also, since God has forgiven us what cost him His son's life, we are also expected to forgive our fellow man. Failing to do this, God would hand us over to tormentors. It is submitted that these tormentors are various types of sicknesses which the devil and his demons can afflict humans with. It is therefore healthy to forgive.

In the Old Testament, God told the Israelites that if they completely obey him, he would put no disease on them.

> *"And said, if thou wilt diligently hearken to the voice of the Lord thy God, and wilt do that which is right in his sight and wilt give ear to his commandments, and keep all his statutes, I will put none of these diseases upon thee which I have brought upon the Egyptians: for I am the Lord*

that healeth thee (Exodus 15:26).

The Jews had a lot of laws given them by God to regulate their conduct. But in the New Testament Jesus left the church with a new commandment: the commandment of love for one another.

> *"A new commandment I give unto you, that ye love one another; as I have loved you, that ye also love one another. By this shall all men know that ye are my disciples, if ye have love one to another" John 13:34-35.*

The apostle Paul in the Book of Roman says that to love is to fulfil the law:

> *"Owe no man anything, but to love one another for he that loveth another hath fulfilled the law" (Romans 13:8).*
> *"Love worketh no ill to his neighbour: therefore love is the fulfilling of the law" (Romans 13:10).*

So, under the New Testament if you love one another, including your enemies, you have fulfilled all the laws of God. Logically, it could be argued that if you love your neighbour including your enemies then one can claim the promises in Exodus 15:20 earlier referred to which is that God would not put any disease on you. He becomes your healer because you have completely obeyed all His commandments by your walking in love.

The Lord turned Job's captivity when he prayed for his friends who had previously accused him unjustly of wrong doing. One of the captivities of Job was ill health. He was made healthy when he prayed for his offending friends.

CHAPTER FOUR

SECRET TO PROTECTION

Never return evil for evil or insult for insult-scolding, tongue-lashing, berating, but on the contrary, blessing - praying for their welfare, happiness and protection and truly pitying and loving them for know that to this you have been called that you may yourself inherit a blessing [from God] - obtain a blessing as heirs, bringing welfare and happiness and protection - 1 Peter 3:9 (Amplified version).

One of the benefits that one inherits from the attitude of never returning evil for evil but blessing your enemies is that you'll be protected by God from harm.

We have noted that the man Job in the Bible displayed such an attitude (see Job 31:29-30). One of those benefits he got from God was that he, his household, and all he had on every side were protected. When God boasted to Satan about the uprightness of Job, Satan confirmed that God had protected him and his household and all that he had:

> *"Then Satan answered the*
> *Lord, and said, Doth Job fear*
> *God for nought,*

> *Hast not thou made an hedge about him and about his house, and about all that he hath on every side? Thou hast blessed the work of his hands and his substance is increased in the land". (Job 1:9-10).*

On the other hand, returning evil for evil and being angry and resentful of your enemies open you up to dangers.

> *"To whom ye forgive anything, I forgive also. For if I forgave anything, to whom I forgave it, for your sakes forgave I it in the person of Christ, lest Satan should get an advantage of us, for we are not ignorant of his devices". (2 Corinthians 2:10-11).*

If you fail to forgive, it's likely that Satan will get advantage over you. He thrives in such atmosphere.

> *"If you are angry, be sure that it is not out of wounded pride or bad temper. Never*

> *go to bed angry – don't give the devil that sort of foothold". (Ephesians 4:26-27 J.B. Philips translation).*
>
> *"If you are angry, don't sin by nursing your grudge. Don't let the sun go down with you still angry – get over it quickly, for when you are angry you give a mighty foothold to the devil" (Ephesians 4:26-27 Living Bible Edition).*

So, retaliating in anger or returning evil for evil in the spirit of anger gives the devil an inroad into your life where he can cause much havoc; whereas not returning evil for evil will give you an inheritance from God which includes protection.

Psalm 91 is a psalm showing the protection that God gives to him that dwelled in the secret place of the Most high. Such a person, says the Psalm, shall abide under the shadow of the Almighty. He will be delivered from the snare of the fowler. God will cover him with His feathers. He says no evil shall befall him, neither shall any plague come nigh his dwelling because He shall give his angels charge over such a person, to keep him in all his ways.

To qualify for all the protection of the Lord specified in Psalm 91, all that a person has to do , according to verse 1, is to dwell in the secret place of the Most high. To dwell in the secret place of the Most high is to dwell in love for your neighbour (including your enemies).

"And we have known and believed the love that God hath to us, God is love: and he that dwelleth in love dwelleth in God, and God in him" – 1 John 4:16.

He that loves his fellow man dwells in the secret place of the Most high and, therefore, entitled to Gods protection as is stated in Psalm 91.

CHAPTER FIVE

THE SECRET TO HAPPINESS

According to the Amplified translation of 1 Peter 3:9, if you don't return evil for evil but rather praying blessings on your enemies then you will inherit blessings of God which includes happiness, welfare and wellbeing.

It has been said that resentment is a non-conductor of spiritual power. It blocks the easy flow of spiritual power from God to the individual.

Proverbs 15:13 (a) says a merry heart maketh a cheerful countenance:

> *Proverbs 15:15 says: "all the days of the afflicted are evil but he that is of a merry heart hath a continual feast."*
> *Proverbs 17:22: a merry heart doeth good like a medicine: but a broken spirit drieth the bones".*

A heart free from resentments is a heart that is merry, which has a continual feast and does good like medicine. As we noted before, Jesus said in the parable of the unforgiving servant that failure to forgive your enemies opens you to affliction. It's even more staggering to realize that if you don't love your enemies by forgiveness, your faith and your prayers won't work.

> *"And when ye stand praying, forgive, if ye have aught against any: that your father also which is in heaven may forgive you your trespasses. But if ye do not forgive, neither will your father which is in heaven forgive your trespasses"* *(Mark 11:25-26).*

Before Jesus made the above statement, He had taught on how to have faith and how to pray effectively in Mark 11:23 & 24. But He qualified his teachings on faith and prayer by saying that for faith and prayer to work you need to forgive anything that you have against anybody.

Moreover when you don't return evil for evil, it means that you are leaving vengeance to God and God really says that He is our avenger. Vengeance is His.

> *"Dearly beloved, avenge not yourselves, but rather give place unto wrath: for it is*

written, vengeance is mine. I will repay, saith the Lord"
Romans 12:19.

In the story of Joseph in the Old Testament, God really brought justice to him. He placed his brothers who tried to kill him and eventually sold him off to slavery at his feet. Thank God Joseph chose to forgive them, instead of paying them back in their own coin. It was a story that had a happy ending.

In my own case, when I was in Higher School at Government College Ughelli, Nigeria, there was a boy who doubled as the school head and the Commanding Officer of the Nigerian Army Cadet Unit attached to the school of which I was also a member. He hated me with a passion for reasons best known to him and he dealt ruthlessly with me.

When we left the school, I went on to study law and didn't hear of him for a long time. Fourteen years later we met in a very strange way. I was now a lawyer and a state prosecutor. He was incarcerated over a case of alleged fraud and his case was assigned to me to handle in Warri. I was awed at the situation. His lawyer pleaded with me that I should help out. Before we could treat his matter I was transferred to another Jurisdiction in Sapele.

Not long after that, his case was refiled in Sapele and assigned to me again to handle. His new Lawyer approached me and pleaded with me to help get him out of jail; I was surprised at the turn of events. The lawyer explained that the bail application first filed in Warri was thrown out and so she decided to file a fresh one in Sapele where coincidentally I was the prosecutor. I helped him out to the best of my ability and of course within the ambits of the law. When he was released from prison we met and he thanked me.

He offered me some presents but I told him that he didn't have to; for what are friends for after all.

In answering the question of what made Joseph great, Chuck Swindoll in his book "*Joseph: from pit to pinnacle*" wrote that Joseph was great because of his attitude, how he responded to difficult circumstances. This he said was the most remarkable thing about him. He quoted the American author Elbert Hubbard as saying that "the final proof of greatness lies in being able to endure (contemptuous treatment) without resentment".

If he was bitter and resentful over the people who had maltreated him the story would not have had a happy ending. He would have ended up tragically with probably a high blood pressure, stomach ulcer, depression or any one of the host of diseases which medical experts attribute to anger, vindictiveness and similar emotional reactions. Joseph found happiness in his life because he was not resentful.

PLEASE LEAVE YOUR COMMENTS
Please take a moment and leave your thoughts about this book on Amazon by clicking here or pasting this link in your browser:
http://amazon.com/author/adigwebooks

Thanks a lot!

OTHER BOOKS BY THE AUTHOR

You can get other exciting books by the author in both paperback and ebook or kindle versions by pasting the following link in your browser: www.amazon.com/author/adigwebooks

Alternatively, you can click any of the titles below to get them on Amazon.

1. Overcoming Depression with the Power of Music
2. The Cost of Answered Prayers

ABOUT THE AUTHOR

Born to Barrister Peter and Mrs Kanwulia Adigwe, attended Obafemi Awolowo University Ile Ife Nigerian and the Nigerian law School Lagos Nigeria. He is a member of the boys scout and a former member of the Nigerian army cadets unit attached to Government College Ughelli. Ben is also a Bible scholar, lawyer and Chartered Mediator and Conciliator. He is also an artist and member of the Full Gospel Business Men Fellowship International. Furthermore, he is a poet and writer, married with kids. a director with the ministry of Justice Asaba and presently deployed to the Delta State Signage and Advertisement Agency where he is presently the functioning Managing Director/ Legal Adviser.

ABOUT THE BOOK

This book examines the price which Christ and other writers of the New Testament say you have to pay to have your prayers answered.

.

www.ingramcontent.com/pod-product-compliance
Lightning Source LLC
Chambersburg PA
CBHW070747240726
48654CB00010B/1200